Osteoa

By
Lynne D M Noble

Copyright 2018 Lynne D M Noble

Independently published

Contents

Acknowledgement

I think that, whenever there is a writer in the house, other family members have to learn a few extra rules. These include remembering to keep quiet just when the writer is holding a number of important concepts in their head and putting up with the masses of paper which appear to land on every conceivable space in the house. In fact, it takes a special sort of person to live with a writer.

This acknowledgement recognises the contribution that my husband, Michael, plays in supporting my working environment.

Dedication

To all sufferers in the hope that this is the answer that you seek

Preface

The definition of pain is that it is a highly unpleasant physical or mental sensation which can be caused by illness, injury or emotional suffering. Some people who are suffering pain may think this is a fairly bald understatement.

There are a few people who do not feel physical pain – congenital analgesia – at all. Most of us will experience pain in its many forms as it has a protective role to play. Pain produces a reflexive retraction from harmful stimuli and protects the body while it heals. Pain, for example, limits the use of the area affected by illness or injury, giving it time to heal.

Osteoarthritis is the most common musculoskeletal condition in older people. According to Arthritis Research UK[1], around one third of people aged 45 years and over in the UK, a total of 8.75 million people, have sought treatment for osteoarthritis. This represents a huge amount of people whose quality of life has diminished to the point where they actively seek help.

---

[1] January 23rd 2013

Osteoarthritis is not an inflammatory arthritis in the way that rheumatoid arthritis is. The breakdown of the cartilage which occurs is not initially due to inflammation although inflammatory processes are involved later.

The pain which afflicts those with osteoarthritis is chronic pain. Chronic pain is often defined as any pain which lasts for more than twelve weeks. It may stem from acute pain which is a normal sensation that alerts us to illness or injury but the sensation of discomfort in chronic pain is entirely different. It is thudding and achy as opposed to the sharp pain of acute pain. Chronic pain is often accompanied by decreased appetite, mood changes, fatigue and, sleep disturbance among others.

When pain receptors are irritated they cause pain. Pain receptors can be found in the joints, skin and internal organs.

There are a number of substances which irritate pain receptors. They are produced by immune system cells and each substance will require a different response in order that it can be managed.

With a little bit of investigation, we can identify the immune system substance which is causing the pain. Then we can deal with it.

However, we also need to look at the underlying processes which initiated the arthritic process in the first place in order to stem any further damage. There are well researched treatments which can alleviate some of the damage in OA as well as the pain. However, these do not form part of current traditional medicine.

This book is intended to inform about the cause of osteoarthritis pain and, just as importantly, what painkillers are most likely to be the optimal response to a specific pain. Further, we will look at some ways of reversing some of the damage which has occurred in the OA process. Damage can be reversed through good and appropriate nutrition. The book will also look at some of the over the counter medications and, some prescription drugs. However, its main intention, when we look at pain relief, is to look at effective analgesia which is not mainstream analgesia.

Alternative pain relief can be maintained until the inclusion of appropriate nutrition has begun to reverse some of the damage to bone and cartilage which is found in osteoarthritis.

Most people have enough knowledge about paracetamol and ibuprofen but do not know about some equally, if not more, effective compounds which can be used as adjunctive pain relief, or as a standalone analgesic. Further these substances often work more quickly, and for longer periods. They also come without some of the side effects of commonly prescribed, or over the counter, medications.

I do not write this book without experience of osteoarthritis. There is a significant family history of osteoarthritis. Further, I fractured a bone in my left foot which was not picked up for five months. Following that injury, I was found to have arthritis in that foot. I was a keen walker and did not appreciate the pain or disability that came with it.

Shortly after, I presented at my GP with painful shoulders. I was found to have arthritis, bursitis and a tear in them. One day, when out in the garden, my knee gave way. It continued to do this with increasing levels of pain. X-rays showed that I had 'mild' arthritis. 'Mild? I couldn't imagine what the full blown variety must feel like.

One of my siblings was, by then, also hobbling with knee arthritis.

I stopped the research I was undertaking on a neurodegenerative disorder and devoted my time to osteoarthritis and pain, grateful that my background was in orthopaedics, initially.

Within two days of following the results of the research and the subsequent advice, I was free from pain in my foot, shoulders and knee. I am now able to walk down stairs without my knee giving way. The stiffness has gone. Neither the pain or stiffness has returned since.

What I have learned is contained in this book. It works because others have followed the advice and had the same results that I had.

This book, is in no way intended to replace the knowledge of your GP but it is a useful and comprehensive source of knowledge for those who wish to further their knowledge of osteoarthritis, how to deal effectively with the pain and start reversing some of the damage of this debilitating disease.

Osteoarthritis – an overview

Osteoarthritis – sometimes referred to as degenerative joint disease - occurs when there is degeneration of the joint cartilage and underlying bone. It is the most common chronic condition of the joints, affecting millions of people. It is more common from middle age onwards -there is good reason for this, which I will explain later. Osteoarthritis causes pain and stiffness, especially in the hip, knee and thumb and small joints of the fingers.

Normal joints have a rubbery material called cartilage which covers the end of each bone. Cartilage is smooth so that it provides a gliding surface for joint motion.

In OA, the cartilage breaks down, causing pain, swelling and problems moving the joint. OA will worsen over time and bone will break down and develop growths called spurs.

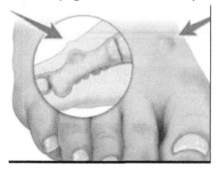

Bone spurs or osteophytes[2]

.

Bits of bone or cartilage may chip off and float around in the joint. This will cause inflammation. During the inflammatory process, chemicals are released which damage the cartilage even further.

Finally, the cartilage wears away and bone rubs against bone. This will create even more joint damage and pain.

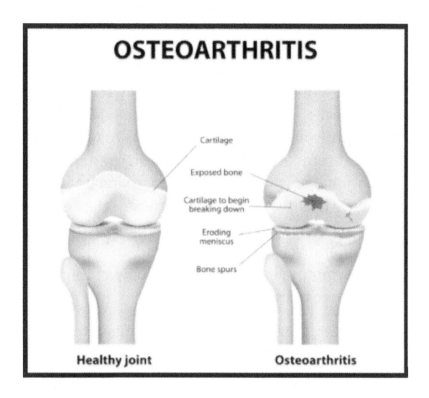

OSTEOARTHRITIS

Cartilage

Exposed bone

Cartilage to begin
breaking down

Eroding
meniscus

Bone spurs

Healthy joint   **Osteoarthritis**

The people who appear to be affected by OA the most are:

- Those from middle-age onwards
- Those who are obese
- Prior joint injury
- Joint overuse

One in two adults will develop symptoms of knee OA during their lives. This may start off as a mild ache, stiffness or the knee giving away without warning. These symptoms may go away but return at a later date. This pattern may continue as the body will be trying to repair itself. Eventually, however, these relapses and repairs will become progressive and degenerative, in nature, without the benefit of the symptomless stages. The only recourse at this stage is knee surgery.

However, knees aren't the only joints affected.

- One in four adults will develop symptoms of hip OA by age 85.

- One in 12 people 60 years or older have hand OA.

- There is a genetic predisposition to osteoarthritis and those with weak thigh muscles are more prone to hip and knee osteoarthritis.

Hip replacement surgery is a procedure in which a doctor surgically removes a painful hip joint with arthritis and replaces it with an artificial hip joint that is generally made from metal and plastic components. Hip surgery is only considered when all other treatment options have failed to provide adequate pain relief.

There are also risks associated with hip replacement – although these do not happen very often, these include:

- Blood clots
- Infection which can occur at the site of the new hip
- Fracture
- Dislocation
- Change in leg length
- loosening

When I was working in orthopaedics it was not unknown for patients in their eighties to benefit from a hip replacement operation. They said it gave them a new lease of life.

However, I said earlier, that there is a reason why those of middle age or over, develop osteoarthritis, without injury, obesity or joint overuse. The reason is that, as we get older, we absorb fewer cartilage building nutrients so cartilage is less able to repair itself. Of course, poor absorption of nutrients, in middle age and beyond, extends far beyond those required for healthy bone and cartilage. However, age-related diseases are not inevitable as long as the necessary building blocks, for repair, are available.

Before we look at how to alleviate the pain, we will examine what we can do to start building healthy cartilage and bone and start reversing the process of osteoarthritis.

We will start this by looking at four remarkable amino acids: glycine, proline, hydroxyproline and arginine that are vital for healthy connective tissue.

Amino acids, antioxidant, anti-inflammatory and pain relieving properties.

The role of glycine

Amino acids are the building blocks of protein and, as such are found in all animal foods Peas, beans and other legumes are also rich sources of amino acids.

Amino acids can be non–essential, that is they can be made in the body, or essential which means they must be taken in through diet. Some amino acids are also said to be conditional which means that normally the body can make them but at times of illness or injury, they may need to be ingested or supplemented.

It would be remiss of me if I did not add glycine as one of the mainstays of the osteoarthritis sufferer's emergency kit. Not only can It can relieve intractable arthritic pain in less than a day but it can continue to employ its anti-inflammatory and

7

analgesic properties if it is taken on a daily basis, in sufficient amounts.

Glycine is the smallest amino acid of the twenty amino acids. Only nine amino acids are classed as essential. Glycine, however, is a non- essential amino acid. This means it is capable of being synthesised from another amino acid, by the body, when needed.

The story should end there but, of course, it doesn't. Our current diets do not support the synthesis of enough glycine to support the growth and repair of healthy bones, muscle tissue, ligaments, tendons and cartilage (which also cushions the spinal discs) required for pain free joints.

> Glycine supports the growth and repair of bones, muscles, ligaments, tendons and cartilage.

Let's look at some more of the actions of this marvellous building block of connective tissue.

Glycine reduces pain

Glycine is an inhibitory amino acid which means that it helps to calm your brain down. This calming influence reduces the sensation of pain. Glycine also helps the absorption of calcium which is good news for those with osteoarthritis and osteoporosis.

Glycine reduces inflammation

Glycine acts directly on cells which are involved in the inflammatory process. It suppresses free radicals which are highly reactive molecules that go around – like an out of control pinball – damaging cells which get in its way. Glycine also suppresses inflammatory cytokines.

Inflammatory cytokines are molecules which are secreted from immune cells like macrophages. These molecules help promote inflammation. Of course, it is the inflammatory processes which cause the pain.

Glycine blocks processes which raise inflammation

Fructose is a type of sugar commonly found in fruit. It has the ability to raise inflammation through a cell signalling molecule called Tumour Necrosis Factor (TNF). Glycine has the ability to block this process and further block another molecule called interleukin 6 which is also involved in the inflammatory process.

Glycine is the major building block of the protein collagen which is found in all connective tissue.

Glycine is required to build strong, connective tissue – in all its forms. This includes the cartilage that is worn away and is notoriously difficult to repair.

Where can glycine be found? Glycine is normally found in many of the foods that we don't eat nowadays. These include:

- Bone broths
- Chicken skin
- Pork scratchings
- Pigs ears
- Tripe
- Organ meats

to name but a few.

In WW1 and WW2 and the immediate post war years, these foods were eaten on a regular basis. Food was scarce and so nothing was wasted. Fish heads were kept to one side to make fish head soup. Chicken bones were stewed slowly until they yielded a clear broth full of goodness. What they all had in common was a protein called gelatin which is the cooked form of collagen.

Gelatin contains 23% of glycine. It plumps up connective tissue making it strong – and in the case of tendons, ligaments and skin – flexible. Bones and muscle are made stronger.

As age progresses, sarcopenia can occur. Sarcopenia is age-related muscle wasting. As muscles waste, joints become weak. They are not up to the job that they were designed to do.

Age related muscle loss – sarcopenia - helps to progress the disabling effects of osteoarthritis.

Normally, the task of building up muscle is left to another amino acid called leucine.

Leucine is an essential amino acid which means that we must get it from dietary sources since our bodies cannot synthesise it. It is called a Branched Chain Amino Acid (BCAA) and is the most abundant amino acid in muscle tissue. Leucine stimulates protein synthesis and muscle tissue. It is therefore a necessary component of healthy joints.

Leucine can be found in all animal foods. There are much smaller amounts in plant sources.

However, the effect of leucine in stimulating the synthesis of muscle tissue is more likely to be seen in younger people. In older people, or in people who have muscle wasting diseases, glycine is the amino acid which helps the synthesis of lean muscle tissue.

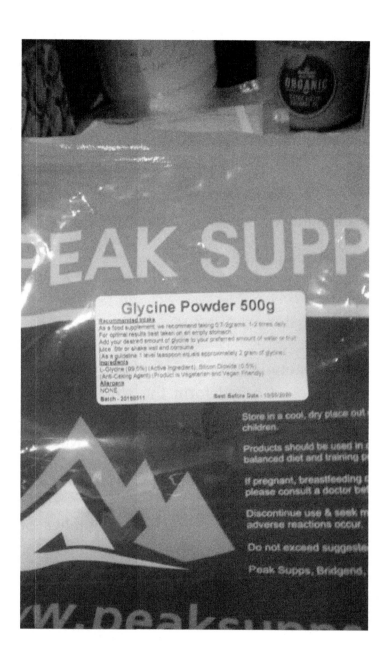

Glycine Powder 500g

Recommended intake
As a food supplement, we recommend taking 0.7-2grams, 1-2 times daily.
For optimal results best taken on an empty stomach.
Add your desired amount of glycine to your preferred amount of water or fruit juice. Stir or shake well and consume.
(As a guideline 1 level teaspoon equals approximately 2 gram of glycine)

Ingredients
L-Glycine (99.5%) (Active Ingredient), Silicon Dioxide (0.5%)
(Anti-Caking Agent) (Product is Vegetarian and Vegan Friendly)

Allergens
NONE

Batch - 20180511   Best Before Date - 10/05/2020

Store in a cool, dry place out
children.

Products should be used in
balanced diet and training p

If pregnant, breastfeeding
please consult a doctor be

Discontinue use & seek m
adverse reactions occur.

Do not exceed suggeste

Peak Supps, Bridgend,

w.peaksu

13

.

Glycine combined with L-theanine (an amino acid found in tea) helps the recovery of tendonitis. Further, as glycine has oestrogen like effects it helps to protect bones.

Glycine can be made from glutamic acid. Glutamic acid is an amino acid which is found in:

- All types of meat
- Dairy
- Eggs
- Fish

The main vegetarian source of glutamic acid is wheat. Pasta and bread form the staple diets of many and should provide all the glycine that we need but, it appears, that many individuals whether on vegan, vegetarian or meat diets may be low in glycine.

Why would this be so? There are a number of reasons including the need to exclude gluten for medical reasons, malnutrition, poor absorption of nutrients (which may be age-related) or something has gone wrong with the mechanism that converts glutamic acid to glycine. This isn't a definitive list.

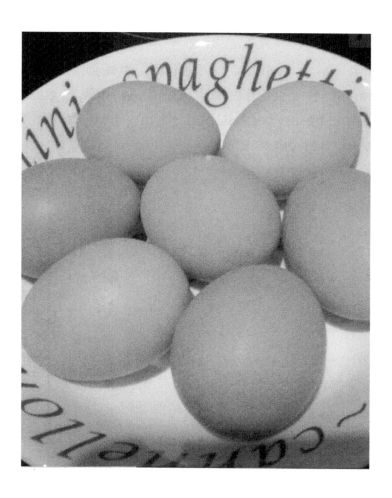

Eggs and pasta are full of glutamic acid which is a precursor to glycine.

When osteoarthritis strikes, I would always recommend changing your diet to include more glycine and I would recommend supplementing with glycine.

Glycine is a white crystalline, sweet tasting substance. It resembles sugar and, as such, is good for sprinkling on cereals and stirring into drinks if you wish to sweeten them.'

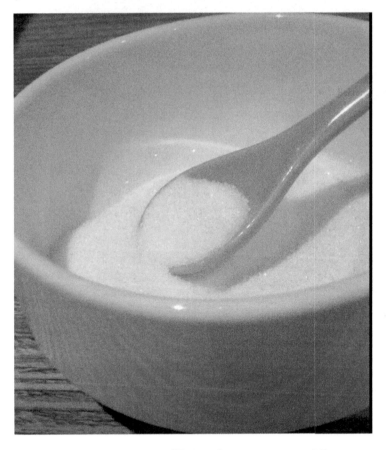

Glycine is a sweet crystalline substance resembling sugar.

I would always recommend that an increase collagen forming amino acids - especially glycine – is incorporated into the diet once the middle twenties are reached. Following this guideline may save many from the back problems, and other osteoarthritic pains, which appear to be rife in older age.

Of course, gelatin is the cooked form of collagen and is used as a setting agent for both savoury and sweet dishes. It can easily be sprinkled over food to increase the glycine/collagen content.

You normally 'bloom' the gelatin before adding it to dishes. This means that you soften it in a little cold water before dissolving it in warmer – but not boiling – liquid.

Gelatin can be seen in 'setting' of bone broth which produces a jelly like stock.

It is also the substance of wine gums and gummy bears. If you are laid up in bed with a bad back, ask for wine gums instead of chocolate!

nentation

10g for two weeks for osteoarthritis followed by 3-5g daily after that.

OR

Gelatin – up to 10g daily, for three months, followed by 5g daily once the pain and stiffness has subsided.

Building up healthy cartilage

Proline is one of those amino acids that nobody seems to have heard about yet its contribution to the health of connective tissue disorders cannot be ignored.

Proline is another non-essential amino acid that has a number of functions including tissue repair and cellular regeneration as well as forming part of the composition of collagen. More proline is produced at times of soft tissue injury, surgery or severe burns.

There is a high demand for proline whenever tissue damage occurs. This also includes damage to bone and cartilage.

The importance of proline in the regeneration of cartilage is a major one. Cartilage is notoriously difficult to regenerate since there are not any blood vessels in cartilage[3] to supply the specialised cells, called chondrocytes, with nutrients.

---

[3] Cartilage is avascular

The nutrients actually diffuse through some quite dense connective tissue which surrounds the cartilage and into the core of the cartilage. Thus repair of cartilage is slow at the best of times and non-existent if a poor diet is followed.

In addition to the above benefits of proline, it keeps muscles and joints flexible, reduces sagging and keeps wrinkles at bay. This is particularly useful for those who spend a lot of time in the sun.

A lack of proline in the diet can be responsible for strains and tears in soft tissue and a poor rate of healing.

Proline also helps to prevent arteriosclerosis – hardening of the arteries – and assists in balancing blood pressure levels.

Further, proline also helps the body break down protein from worn out cells in the body. The end result of this degradation is then used to create new healthy cells. Proline is also required to form hydroxyproline. Hydroxyproline is yet another amino acid which is a major component of the protein, collagen.

Good sources of proline are: egg yolks, grass fed meats, organ meats – for example, liver and kidney, bone broth and gelatin. Many of these simply do not form part of our diet anymore.

If we look at the above foods in the light of our current eating preferences, grass fed meats, organ meats, bone broth and gelatin are foods of the past. Further, eggs have been demonised as being a contributory factor to high cholesterol levels. They may well do, but high cholesterol levels are associated with a number of healthy states which will be the subject of a later book.

Proline is synthesised from glutamic acid which is another amino acid. As long as the diet is sufficient in glutamic acid then there should be sufficient proline. However, in cases of connective tissue disorder, it would be helpful to supplement with proline since we are less able to synthesise substances as we age. Be guided by the dosage instructions, which accompanies proline, on its packaging.

It is harder to find sources of proline than glycine and it does tend to be more expensive than glycine. However, it is worth sourcing, even if it is a one off purchase in order to see how effective supplementing with proline is in ameliorating osteoarthritis.

Glutamic acid, from which proline is made, is found in all types of animal protein: eggs, meat, fish and cheese, for example. It does not usually need to be supplemented. However, if the diet needs supplementing at times of illness or advancing age then whey protein is an easily digestible source of all the essential amino acids.

About 30% of the protein in wheat is made from glutamic acid.

Vegetarian sources of proline include:

- cabbage
- peanuts
- soy products
- watercress
- asparagus
- white mustard seeds.

Hydroxyproline

Hydroxyproline is a major component of the protein collagen. It helps to prevent fine lines and wrinkles found in aged or sun damaged skin. Rat studies found that there was an increasing effect of an oral intake of L-hydroxyproline on the soluble collagen content of skin.

In this study[4] either 0.5 or 1g/kg of hydroxyproline (Hyp) was given to rats. After 2 weeks, administration of Hyp the soluble collagen content of the skin had increased.

This suggested that oral hydroxyproline, improved collagen metabolism.

Any defect in collagen synthesis can lead to a number of effects such as easy bruising, breakdown of connective tissue, internal bleeding, thin walled blood vessels. As can be seen from the table below, without an adequate supply of vitamin C, then the

---

[4] https://www.ncbi.nlm.nih.gov/pubmed/22790956

synthesis of collagen, from hydroxyproline, cannot occur.

Vitamin C is a water soluble vitamin. It is found in fresh fruit and vegetables. It is easily destroyed by heat and sunlight. It is a powerful anti-inflammatory vitamin.

The recommended daily allowance is 30mg daily which is the amount found in a medium size orange. However, in connective tissue disorders, I would be recommending much higher amounts. There are some dissolvable vitamin C tablets (ascorbic acid) which are generally a reasonable price. They can be found in supermarkets. They contain 1000mg of vitamin C. About half a tablet daily can be taken for a couple of weeks, 100mg for another two weeks and then 30-100mg daily following this.

Vitamin C can cause diarrhoea. When it does this it is referred to as 'bowel tolerance.' When this occurs then this is the highest dose that can be consumed and your dose should not exceed this.

As vitamin C is a water soluble tablet, any excess not required by the body, is simply lost through urine.

There is little point in increasing vitamin C though, in order to treat osteoarthritis, if the proline content of food has not increased too; both are required to make hydroxyproline.

Diagram showing chain of events in forming collagen from glutamic acid.

Glutamic Acid

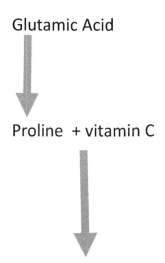

Proline + vitamin C

hydroxyproline + glycine (from serine) and arginine

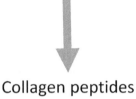

Collagen peptides

Vegetarian and non-vegetarian sources of hydroxyproline:

Non-vegetarian:

- meat,
- pigs trotters
- monkfish
- eggs
- shark cartilage
- milk and other dairy products

Vegetarian sources of hydroxyproline:

- carob seeds
- Alfalfa sprouts
- Citrus fruits (or anything high in vitamin C)

- Vegetable foods high in vitamin c (peppers, cabbage, parsley

Non citrus fruits such as banana also help in the synthesis of hydroxyproline.

Now that we have looked at glycine, proline and hydroxyproline, we will turn our attention to the fourth major component of collagen. This is the amino acid, arginine.

Arginine

Arginine is an essential amino acid which means that it has to be obtained from the diet. It is unusual in that, in the body, it is known to change into nitric oxide. Nitric oxide is a powerful neurotransmitter. It helps blood vessels to relax thereby improving circulation.

Arginine is also a component of many connective tissues and supports the production of collagen. Further, arginine assists with the growth of osteoblasts which are the cells which form bone mass.

A study[5] from 2002 showed that arginine was important for bone health since a deficiency of this amino acid was implicated in osteoporosis.

A standard daily dose for arginine has not yet been agreed but most people ingest about 23 grams per day.

Good food sources of arginine are:

- turkey (one turkey breast contains about 16gm)
- pork loin (approximately 13gm)
- chicken
- peanuts
- soybeans
- dairy

When we are looking at the foods which contribute to healthy connective tissue then time and again the humble peanut turns up.

If you are a fan of peanuts - and peanut butter - then this is to your advantage but, of course,

---

[5] https://www.aminoacid-studies.com/areas-of-use/arthritis-andosteoporosis.html

there are many people who appear to have developed an allergy to this food. Allergies also appear rife in connective tissue disorders so those with connective tissue disorders cannot always benefit from this nutritious food. However, the point that needs underlining is that peanuts are another food which were very popular during the war, and immediate post war period. They appear to have fallen out of popularity along with many other foods which promote the synthesis of healthy connective tissue.

During the war years, nothing was wasted – even pig trotters could contribute to a warming gelatinous soup if they were slowly simmered for some time.

If a return to some of the recipes which were part of the daily diet in the 1940's and 1950's does not appeal – although I think you should give them a try

- then there are plenty of collagen powders online which are made from dried fish scales and chicken feet, among others, which you could add to shakes, omelettes or soups. There are also supplements of collagen available which are also convenient for those who do not enjoy cooking. 10-15g daily should suffice for those who have poor connective tissue. Nevertheless, bone broth is still an essential for good connective tissue health. Add some garlic and onion to it and you are increasing the amount of methionine – another amino acid – which is required to build good cartilage.

Methionine is a sulphur containing amino acid. It is an essential amino acid and therefore must be obtained from food. Methionine helps to make SAM-e (S- Adenosyl Methionine) which is used in the production of creatine. This is an important substance for cellular energy. However, the importance of SAM-e in osteoarthritis can be seen in its superior anti-inflammatory effects.

A 2004 study[6] undertaken by the University of California, found SAM-e equal to the prescription drug celecoxib (Celebrex) and a 2009 study[7] found

[6] https://www.ncbi.nlm.nih.gov/pubmed/15102339

it comparable to the NSAID nabumetone. Further studies[8] – that included both in vitro and animal studies have shown that SAM-e can stimulate the production of cartilage. This is a critical process required for reversing arthritis.

Eggs, fish and meat contain good amounts of the amino acid, methionine. Whenever supplemental methionine is taken it is judicious to take a supplement of vitamin B complex. They work together to keep you healthy.

MSM powder is normally dissolved in water. It tastes a little bitter so it can either be dissolved in orange juice or a sweet sucked immediately after it has been swallowed. Be guided by the instructions on the packaging. MSM also comes in capsules and tablet form. It is purely a matter of personal preference which is take.

The general 'rule' for the daily allowance of MSM is to supplement with 19mg for every kilogram of body weight.

---

[7] https://www.ncbi.nlm.nih.gov/pubmed/20110025
[8] https://www.ncbi.nlm.nih.gov/pubmed/18464034

Here is a recipe, for bone broth, which will help increase the intake of those components required for good collagen synthesis.

Bone broth

Some people may think it is a lot of work making their own stock from bones and fish head and storing it in the freezer but it is definitely worth doing. The alternative is to use those stock cubes which contain mainly salt, a little yeast and some animal fat. The gelatin is absent and it is this we are trying to put back into the diet.

The stock will keep well for a month or so, in the freezer, but I never find it lasts that long. I always seem to have some on the go. I am quite happy throwing some bones into the slow cooker with some herbs, garlic and onion, waiting until it cools before transferring it to a jam jar ready to place into the freezer.

I leave about a one-inch space to allow for expansion at the top of the jar.

When I eventually thaw the stock, it is entirely up to me what other vegetables I throw into it. You can add white wine to white meat, and fish stocks. and red wine to the darker meats and oilier fishes. I don't use alcohol at all but some people want to add it to just about everything. Really, all you need is a little motivation and a lot of imagination to produce your own range of tasty medicines.

In the words of the old adage:

Let food be your medicine

Taurine – a good all round amino acid

Taurine is another amino acid that deserves a great deal of attention when it comes to reversing osteoarthritis. It is an amino acid which is not – unusually – used in protein synthesis. It is often referred to as a **non-essential** amino acid or sometimes as a **conditionally essential** amino acid.

Taurine forms a major part of the diet of the long lived Japanese in Okinawa where living well, to over a century, is not unusual.

Taurine plays an important role in many vital biological processes which also include the processes found in the immune system.

When we examine acute inflammation we can see that it is a response by the innate immune system to harmful stimuli such as:

- Irritants

- Damaged cells
- Infection
- Cancer cells

The innate immune system is the immunity that you are born with. This system has a general response to harmful stimuli. It is really the first line of defence for damage and diseased cells. The cells of the innate immune system kill infection and clear away any debris that is left after their assault on the invader. Without this 'clearing away' then the healing process could not occur.

The difficulty is that inflammation can continue long after the original injury has healed. Cells continue pouring damaging chemicals into and around the area which has long since healed. This naturally damages healthy tissue. This is the beginning of chronic inflammation. Chronic inflammation serves no useful purpose at all since it is not a 'healing' inflammation. Chronic inflammation is painful and destructive.

Taurine is helpful in osteoarthritis in a number of ways. It helps to maintain calcium homeostasis. It has antioxidant activity and therefore neutralises the free radicals which dash around damaging any cells which get in its way. Taurine has been shown to reach a particularly high concentration in tissues exposed to higher levels of inflammatory cells. Taurine is known to detoxify hypochlorous acid at the site of inflammation.

Anyone with chronic inflammation should be taking taurine as a supplement.

Hypochlorous acid   a substance produced by the kamikaze neutrophil – a small, white fearless cell which drops this potent acid on invading infections, when it is activated. Of course, hypochlorous acid is able to damage normal cells, if it gets out of control. This is where taurine is invaluable as it helps in attenuating programmed cell death (apoptosis). It does this by reacting with the hypochlorous acid to produce two much less toxic substances known as taurine chloramine and taurine bromamine.

Taurine + hypochlorous acid = taurine chloramine +/or   taurine bromamime

As well as exerting anti-inflammatory properties, these two products of the reaction of taurine with hypochlorous acid also have antimicrobial effects. This is good news if the inflammatory processes are provoked by an infective agent.

Most people will be deficient in taurine. As it is found in animal foods, it is highly likely that vegetarians and vegans will be deficient in this wonder molecule. However, even meat eaters are likely to be deficient in taurine. The average diet contains just a mere 59mg whereas we should be ingesting approximately 1000 -1500mg daily. Ageing clearly does not help as individuals tend to eat less, and absorb less of the nutrients, in the food that they do eat.

Taurine can even help in individuals where obesity is accelerating arthritic changes. Firstly, taurine helps with insulin sensitivity.

You may be wondering what insulin sensitivity has to do with osteoarthritis but insulin sensitivity is a mechanism that determines how efficiently your body uses insulin.

If individuals have low insulin sensitivity, then they have a greater chance of developing metabolic diseases such as diabetes.

Greater insulin sensitivity helps individuals to lose weight. Cells becomes more effective in using carbohydrates for energy. This helps you lose weight because your cells are able to use the energy you take in through diet. Further, the increased energy which arises from this process, may mean that an individual takes more exercise.

However, we also need to examine taurine in the light of inflammation producing fat cells and taurine's ability to fight obesity. Taurine was found, when taken at 3g daily, in a study[9] of overweight or obese individuals, to produce significant weight loss over a period of seven weeks. Even a small amount of weight reduction alleviates the progression and pain of osteoarthritis especially in the hips and knees which tend to be most affected as they are the main weight bearing joints.

Taurine must surely deserve pride of place in a cocktail of supplements which are designed to remedy the underlying causes of osteoarthritis and reverse the disease.

Methionine, cartilage and arthritis.

---

[9] http://www.infinitelabs.com/what-is-taurine/

Professor and Dr Klaus Miehlke was classed as the leading expert on bone diseases in Germany. He has argued that in cases of joint or cartilage disease, it is of the utmost importance that the human body receives the cartilage-forming substances in sufficient quantities. He states that a healthy diet cannot provide this and recommends supplements which contain cartilage-forming substances.

Methionine is one such cartilage forming substance. It is an essential amino acid which means it must be taken in from the diet.

Methionine donates sulphur and joint cartilage requires sulphur for its creation. Tests have shown that cartilage in healthy individuals contains around three times more sulphur than in patients who suffer from arthritis. Patients who have arthritis are advised to supplement with methionine and the B vitamins to optimise the results.

Methionine has particular importance in three main areas

- it stimulates the cartilage cells to create more cartilaginous tissue

- contains anti- inflammatory properties

- has an analgesic effect

Dietary sources of methionine include onions, garlic, eggs, meat, fish, sesame seeds, nuts. Most fruit and vegetables contain little methionine although sulphur containing compounds are found in Brussels sprouts and broccoli.

Arginine helps create new bone therefore it is particularly useful for those with a propensity towards osteoporosis.

Arginine supports the production of collagen, which is a protein that is a basic component of connective tissues, like cartilage. It also supports the growth of osteoblasts. These are cells which form new bone.

When a deficiency of arginine occurs it can cause osteoporosis. Studies have shown that arginine in combination with other amino acids supported the growth of osteoblasts[10] It was therefore recommended that the administration of amino acids belonged to all osteoporosis treatments. Arginine is found in all animal foods, soybeans, peanuts, walnuts and pumpkin seeds.

[10] Ursini, F. & Pipicelli, G. (2009) *Nutritional Supplementation for Osteoarthritis,* Alternative and Complementary Therapies, Volume 15, issue 4, (pp. 173-177)

Minerals and vitamins required to repair and reverse the damage found in osteoarthritis

Manganese

Please don't confuse this with magnesium - the only thing that these minerals have in common is that they are extremely good at relieving the pain of osteoarthritis.

Most people know little, if anything about manganese. It is a trace mineral which means that your body only needs it in tiny amounts. However, it is still an essential nutrient which can be found in seeds, whole grains, legumes, beans nuts, leafy green vegetables and tea.

Manganese is essential for bone health including the development and maintenance of bone. When it is combined with zinc, copper and calcium, it does support bone mineral density. Research has shown that it helps reduce spinal bone loss in older women.

A study found that in women with weak bones, when the above nutrients were taken in addition to vitamin D, magnesium and boron, it helped improve bone mass. [11]

The antioxidant enzyme superoxide dismutase (SOD) is one of the most important enzymes in your body. It is partially composed from manganese.

SOD helps neutralise free radicals which can damage cells. It can do this by breaking down superoxide -which is a very large and damaging free radical - into smaller ones which won't damage your cells. There is evidence that SOD is useful as a therapeutic agent for inflammatory disorders. Another study showed that out of 93 people with osteoarthritis, 52% reported symptom improvements after 4 and 6 months of taking a manganese, glucosamine and chondroitin supplement. However, this only appeared to work on the less severe types of osteoarthritis.

---

[11] https://www.ncbi.nlm.nih.gov/pubmed/15658548

Selenium is an essential trace element which most people are deficient in. Our impoverished soil is selenium deficient which means that our food will also be deficient in this mineral.

Scientists have found that for every additional tenth of a part per million of selenium in volunteers' bodies, there was a 15-20% decrease in their risk of knee osteoarthritis.[12]

Those who had less of the trace mineral than normal in their systems faced a higher risk of the degenerative condition in one and both knees. The severity of their arthritis related to how deficient in selenium they were.

Good food sources of selenium are:

- Brewer's yeast
- Garlic
- Liver
- Eggs

---

[12] https://www.sciencedaily.com/releases/2005/11/051114112959.htm

Animal sources of selenium are much higher than those from plants. It is interesting to note that deficiencies of selenium can result in premature ageing and nerve disorders. Two brazil nuts can supply the daily recommended amount but, as selenium is toxic, it is advised that the recommended daily allowance of 200 micrograms is not exceeded.

Eggs are a good source of selenium.

The beauty of boron

Boron is a trace element which is required in the body in tiny amounts but any deficiency will have serious side effects. These include:

- Neural malfunction
- Osteoporosis
- Arthritis
- Hormone imbalance
- Hyperthyroidism
- Abnormal metabolism of calcium

A number of studies in both controlled animal and human studies have provided evidence for the use of boron as a safe and effective treatment for osteoarthritis. These studies have shown that in areas where boron intake is greater than, or equal to one milligram daily, the estimated incidence of arthritis ranges from 20 -70%. In areas where boron intake is usually 3mg to 10mg daily, the estimated incidence of arthritis ranges from 0-10% which is significantly lower.

The boron concentration was found to be lower in the femur heads, bones and synovial fluid of patients with osteoarthritis compared with individuals who did not have osteoarthritis.

Boron has also been found to downregulate enzymes involved in the inflammatory response.

In the severe OA group, average pain reduction was 47.9% at 4 weeks and 64.5% at 8 weeks. In the first 4 weeks, 40% of subjects with severe OA reduced or eliminated their analgesic use (ibuprofen). By week 8, 75% had quit using their NSAID medication (ibuprofen). Joint rigidity disappeared in one half of the severe OA patients in the first 4 weeks. In the remaining one-half of the severe OA, joint rigidity decreased significantly, an average rigidity reduction of 50% of severe OA subjects at 4 weeks and in 62.5% at 8 weeks.

More recently, calcium fructoborate 110mg x d, which provides approximately 3mg of boron 2X daily or 6mg daily, was shown to improve knee discomfort within the first 14 days of treatment.

There is an upper limit (UL) of 20mg daily and effects of boron do not appear to occur until a minimum of 3mg daily is taken.

Good sources of boron per 100g are:

- Raisins 4.51mg
- Almonds 2.82mg
- Hazelnuts 77mg
- Dried apricots 2.11mg
- Peanut butter 1.92mg
- Brazil nuts 1.72mg
- Walnuts 1.63mg
- Red kidney beans 1.4mg
- Prunes 1.18mg
- Cashew nuts (raw) 1.15mg
- Dates 1.08mg
- Chickpeas 0.71mg
- Lentils 0.74mg
- Peaches 0.52mg

Although good sources of boron are brazil nuts, these contain selenium which is toxic if more than two are eaten daily. Therefore, do not eat more than two brazil nuts daily.

Boron healthy recipe

Ingredients

- Two tablespoons peanut butter
- Coconut milk
- Grated apple
- Grated fresh ginger
- Cooked lentils
- Curry powder

Method

Place all the ingredients in a pan – apart from the fresh ginger - and cook through. Sometimes, it helps to leave the cooked mixture in a cool place to allow the flavours to develop. Warm through and serve with fresh grated ginger and, if you like, some toasted almonds.

The above recipe will address a number of pain pathways. For example, lentils are full of tryptophan which is a precursor to serotonin which also inhibits pain.

If the meal is served with pineapple juice it will also inhibit bradykinin which has an inflammatory role.

The role of Magnesium

Along with calcium, magnesium is required to build strong healthy bones. Most people do obtain enough calcium in their diets and are aware of the sources of calcium. However, ask people about magnesium and they are less sure what it does and which foods you would obtain it from.

Magnesium is necessary to make strong, firm bones. It makes teeth less likely to decay, too. It is necessary for the conversion of vitamin D into its active form. Without sufficient magnesium in the diet, a deficiency can lead to a syndrome known as vitamin D resistance.

Vitamin D is required to absorb calcium and phosphorus into the bones. Without adequate magnesium   this process could not occur resulting in weak bones.

In a rat model of osteoarthritis, a deficiency of dietary magnesium was demonstrated to enhance the amount of cartilage damage.[13]

Magnesium also helps to reduce pain. We shall look at this later as well as learn of the sources of magnesium.

It would be remiss of me not to say that if someone is taking diuretics or laxatives, that there is a good chance that they will be magnesium deficient. There is an increased chance of magnesium loss when these medications are taken.

Recommended Daily Allowance is 500mg.

13

https://www.ncbi.nlm.nih.gov/pmc/articles/PMC2265739/

Vitamin D

Approximately 80% of the world population are deficient in this vitamin which is required for strong bones as well as regulating inflammation. It is one of the most difficult of vitamins to take in sufficient quantities through the diet. Foods containing vitamin D are limited and what foods there are do not contain great amounts. As we get older we are less likely to absorb the nutrients from our diet. Vitamin D is no different so increasing age is a risk factor for a deficiency of vitamin D.

Most of our vitamin D is taken in through the action of the sun's rays on the skin but even this process becomes less efficient as we age.

Supplementation of 2000 IU's is recommended daily.

This should be the active form D3 rather than the inactive form, D2. The latter requires a number of steps to be converted to the active form. As age progresses, the conversion process is likely to be less effective.

Dietary sources of vitamin D are irradiated mushrooms, eggs and oily fish. However, supplementation of vitamin D should only be taken in conjunction with adequate vitamin K2. Vitamin K2 is found in fermented foods including hard cheese and kefir.

Acute and Chronic Pain

Be patient and tough; someday this pain will be useful to you
    Ovid

To begin to understand pain - and which treatment is best for a specific pain - there are a number of concepts which need to be understood. The first of these is understanding the difference between acute and chronic pain.

Acute pain is caused by the activation of pain receptors throughout the body from stimuli. The pain is not diffuse – which can happen with chronic pain. The location of acute pain is instantly known and it is caused by tissue damage. It has a set purpose – that of alerting you to the injury and protecting you from further injury. An example of acute pain is the pain which is immediately felt on standing on a nail.

With chronic pain, the reason for the pain may not be known; there may be no known prior illness or injury. Chronic pain may vary in intensity without any apparent cause. The original injury, if it is known appears to have healed yet the pain continues

Sometimes chronic pain occurs as a result of unresolved inflammation as happens in the later stages of osteoarthritis. It may also occur due to damage to the nervous system as in neuropathic pain (traumatic injury, stroke and post-herpetic neuralgia and multiple sclerosis) and unknown precipitating factors such as is seen in Fibromyalgia.

While acute pain is short lived, chronic pain is seen as pain which continues for longer than twelve weeks. It appears to serve no adaptive purpose.

Chronic pain

As we have just learned chronic pain is pain which lasts for longer than twelve weeks. It is more of a dull, thudding background pain in contrast to acute pain, which is sharp and sudden.

There are more medications which act on chronic pain than there are for acute pain. With chronic pain there is often no obvious immediate injury, which could account for it and the underlying cause is entirely different from that found in acute pain.

The role of microglia in pain

The activation of microglia which are cells in the central nervous system are responsible for chronic pain [14] Microglia are the macrophages (scavengers) of the central nervous system. Studies have shown that spinal microglia were activated in response to injury of peripheral nerves.

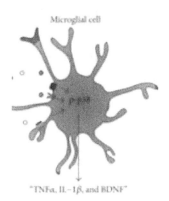

Microglial cell

"TNFα, IL−1β, and BDNF"

---

[14] theconversation.com/what-causes-chronic-pain-microglia-might-be-to-blame-6173

Spinal microglia are activated when damage to peripheral nerves happens. However, glycine, which we have already come across, inhibits the activation of microglia, thus reducing the potential for pain.

When minocycline (an antibiotic which can cross the blood brain barrier) was administered to rats it was found to prevent pain. Minocycline inhibits microglia and other cells - such as astrocytes - from 'cross talking' with neurons. It has been firmly established that this cross talk is necessary for the development of chronic pain.

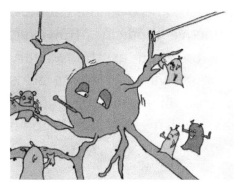

[15] **Microglia cross talk with brain cells this is how they develop and maintain chronic pain.**

Sometimes **breakthrough pain** occurs between the administration of regular

[15] http://blog.donders.ru.nl/?p=4862&lang=en

scheduled painkillers. In some cases, the dose of painkiller can be increased but, in some cases, this is not possible without being harmful.

Some people may turn to alternative medicine to alleviate breakthrough pain. The types of alternative medicine may include aromatherapy, acupuncture or massage.

Some amino acids have pain relieving properties

Many amino acids have powerful anti-inflammatory and analgesic properties. They can be used alongside prescribed, and over the counter, medications as an adjunctive medicine. However, they can just as easily be used as the primary medication. The therapeutic value of amino acids will be discussed in more detail later in this book as will other substances which deal with pain effectively.

Some antidepressants have pain relieving properties

Antidepressants work by increasing the body's own pain fighting resources. They do this by inhibiting pain signalling at the level of the spinal cord. That is, they dampen pain signals. There are a number of substances which can be used without prescription which do exactly the same thing but often without the side effects which tend to go hand in hand with prescription medication. We will look at these in more detail later.

Some people are very stoic and do not want to take painkillers. This is their right. However, all pain as a result of injury will create a neurological pathway where it is registered. This will become more entrenched the longer an injury remains unhealed. Further, even when the injury has healed and no longer presents a problem, there is still the matter of the pathway in the brain which will still register pain. This is where pain is felt, in the brain.

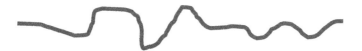

The pain pathway in the brain which registered the pain of an injury, still remains even when the original injury heals.

Therefore, it is of great importance that pain is addressed as soon as is possible. The stoic among us, who do not resort to painkillers, may be troubled with long standing pain as a result of the neurological pathways which have 'captured' the pain resulting from the original injury. This pain can continue long after the injury has healed.

It takes a long time to lose a memory. We only have to smell a whiff of tobacco to be taken back to when we were a child watching as grandad lit his pipe.

Chronic pain is also slow pain. It originates internally. It is poorly localised. The pain is diffuse and the origin cannot be firmly established by the patient. It may radiate out so that it is hard to pinpoint exactly where it is coming from.

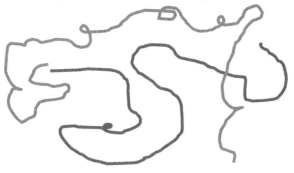

Slow pain is difuse. It is difficult to ascertain the origin of the pain.

Opioids work very well on slow pain. Local anaesthetics block all nerve transmission and also work well on slow pain as well as acute pain.

The impulse from the slow pain is distributed diffusely in the brain and, as such, each area in the brain elicits a different response. This explains why slow pain can cause a wide range of symptoms such as

- Sleeplessness
- Mood changes
- Restlessness
- Loss of appetite

Case History

Linda was 53 when her knee just appeared to 'give' one day when she was walking down some stone steps. Luckily, she was holding onto some handrails at the time otherwise, as she stated, she would have gone flying. Linda did not report any pain and, after about a week, this tendency for her knee to give went. A few months later, this

pattern repeated itself only this time she reports feeling a slight ache at the front of her knee. This, too, disappeared after a couple of weeks and she thought no more of it until some weeks later she found herself struggling to get on the bus as her knee kept giving. The pain, by this point, had increased and was beginning to get her down. The steady aching had already begun to keep her awake and she admitted that she was feeling more and more irritable.

Linda went to her GP who ordered an x-ray for her. This found that Linda has mild arthritis. Linda was informed that she should lose weight and take anti-inflammatories. This appears to be working at the
moment.

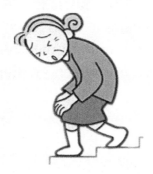

Knees which are osteoarthritic are likely to give away without warning.

Substances released inside the body which contribute to pain.

Although we tend to think of chemical pain receptors being stimulated by chemicals in our environment, there are a good number of chemicals which originate in our body which are released in response to inflammation and trauma among other stimuli.

Redness and heat which occur at the site of injury are due to increased blood flow to the site of inflammation. The swelling is caused by an accumulation of fluid. This presses on nerve endings causing pain. Pain is also due to the release of substances that stimulate pain receptors or the lack of substances which would help ameliorate pain.

Some of these substances are
- Potassium ions
- Lactic acid
- Bradykinins
- Prostaglandins
- Histamine
- Serotonin
- Enkephalins

Pharmacological increase of peripheral potassium ion channel activity consistently alleviated pain in laboratory tests. This simply means that the more potassium ions that were shunted down potassium channels in the cell walls the more that pain was likely to be alleviated.

This action, of course, would depend on there being enough potassium in the diet in the first place. Potassium losses through the use of diuretics and/or laxatives could increase the potential for pain. Further, some people just do not have a diet which incorporates enough potassium into it.

Prunes, dates, raisins, bananas and tomatoes are just some food items which are rich in potassium.

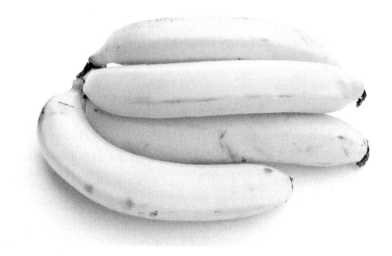

Lactic acid is the acid which causes muscle pain after heavy exercise. It builds up and irritates nerve endings. When our muscles are sore we rub them which stimulates different nerves not connected with transmitting pain from sore muscles.

Sometimes, sore muscles are a result of microscopic tears in muscle after heavy exercise.

Bradykinin is released in response to tissue injury. It is implicated in chronic pain.

Some bradykinin inhibitors which suppress trauma-induced swelling are:
- Bromelain
- Aloe
- Polyphenols found in red wine and green tea
- Apple

When there are microscopic tears, ibuprofen and other NSAIDS's should not be taken immediately, nor should warm baths. Both can cause bleeding from the microscopic tears, increasing pain.

Athletes sit in baths of ice cold water after major exercise to reduce any pain and damage caused by these tiny tears. The same rule applies to sprains and strains which should be treated initially with cold compresses. After two or three days when any microscopic bleeding into the tissue is likely to have resolved then alternate hot and cold compresses will help healing substances flow to the site of injury and assist in removing toxic waste products.

When we encounter painful stimuli, chemicals called prostaglandins are released alongside them. They increase the sensitivity of pain receptors.

Why we need copper

Lysil oxidase is a copper enzyme that is involved in the cross linking of elastin and collagen. As such it is necessary for proper collagen formation and maintenance. As we have now established that cartilage and bone both need collagen to form properly then the value of sufficient copper in the diet can be seen.

When a copper deficiency occurs then damaged connective tissue cannot be replaced. Further, the collagen that makes up the scaffolding of the bone cannot be formed leading to a condition known as osteoporosis. As osteoporosis is a condition normally associated with older age then it could be argued that poorer absorption of nutrients, and less attention to a nutritious diet, could account for a deficiency. High levels of zinc and vitamin C can also deplete copper over time.

Foods which contain copper include:

- Liver
- Oysters
- Nuts and seeds
- Lobster
- Dark leafy greens
- Dark chocolate

The recommended dietary allowance is 900mcg daily. However, a word of caution is required here – a deficiency or excess of copper can have negative side effects so supplementation is not recommended unless under medical supervision.

My recommendation is that every individual with a connective tissue disorder, such as osteoarthritis, look at the composition of their diet to ascertain if it contains enough foods that contain copper and to include them if they are sparse.

Other signs of a copper deficiency include:

- abnormal skin and hair pigmentation
- iron deficient anaemia

- poorly functioning immune system resulting in bacterial infections
- poor memory and lack of creative thinking.

The following foods are excellent sources of copper:[16]

	Amount	RDI
Beef liver, cooked	1 oz (28 g)	458%
Oysters, cooked	6	133%
Lobster, cooked	1 cup (145 g)	141%
Lamb liver, cooked	1 oz (28 g)	99%
Squid, cooked	3 oz (85 g)	90%

---

[16] https://www.healthline.com/nutrition/copper-deficiency-symptoms#section11

Dark chocolate	3.5 oz bar (100 g)	88%
Oats, raw	1 cup (156 g)	49%
Sesame seeds, roasted	1 oz (28 g)	35%
Cashew nuts, raw	1 oz (28 g)	31%

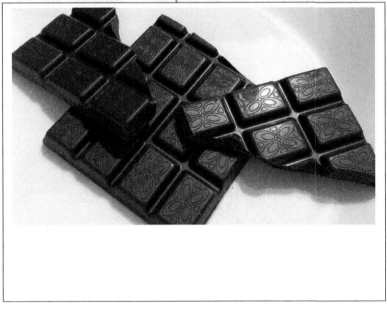

Dark chocolate contains useful amounts of copper

Pain Relievers

How does capsaicin block pain?

Pain receptors become exhausted very quickly if an ointment containing capsaicin is used. In a similar vein, a meal containing cayenne peppers or red and green chilli peppers is high in capsaicin and will also help to exhaust pain signals. This is good news for those who enjoy spicy diets.

Non-steroidal anti-inflammatory drugs (NSAIDS) work well for this type of pain as they reduce the effect of prostaglandins. They act on the peripheral nervous system.

Paracetamol also works well on this type of pain but paracetamol operates in the central nervous system.

Sometimes, when you go to the GP, they will suggest that you take paracetamol and ibuprofen (NSAID) for pain. Taken this way their ability to reduce pain exceeds the ability of the sum of each separate painkiller, when added together.

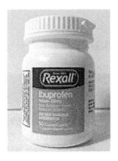

Ibuprofen reduces the effect of prostaglandins, reducing the sensitivity of pain receptors.

Antihistamines can also be useful in inhibiting pain. Most people associate antihistamines with allergic reactions such as hay fever and urticaria. They have never considered them as useful drugs which can help to reduce pain levels.

Histamine is a vasoactive amine which has an important role in the early acute inflammatory response. It is stored in the granules of mast cells, basophils and platelets which are cells which belong to the immune system.

Histamine is released from cells by stimuli which include acute inflammation. Histamine increases vasodilation - that is it widens blood vessels. It also makes them more permeable. Histamine is a chemical mediator and brings immune system substances to the site of injury. They cause swelling and pain.

Diagram showing how injury leads to inflammation

Injury   **releases histamine**
                             which releases

Bradykinins,   prostaglandins   and   other
inflammatory mediators

Some patients ca   ID's such as
ibuprofen or vari   They may be
hypersensitive to ibuprofen or be on medication
such as methotrexate where such anti-
inflammatories are not recommended.   In these
cases, an alternative painkiller should be sought to
be taken alongside paracetamol.   Some antihistamines have sedating effects and have

particular use if pain is disrupting sleep. Of course, the non- sedating, newer type antihistamines can be used during the day.

Why do opioids work on pain?

The brain has a natural brake on pain. Once a pain stimulus hits the brain, the brain leaps into action and sends a signal back to the spinal cord to reduce the pain signal.

Two important molecules in this process are serotonin and encephalin.

Serotonin is a chemical that nerve cells produce which allows messages to be passed between nerve cells. It is mostly found in the digestive system but it can be found in blood platelets and serum, too.

The messages it passes along are related to mood, sexual desire, memory and learning, appetite, sleep and temperature regulation among others. Serotonin also has a major role to play in modulating pain perception. Serotonergic drugs are use in the treatment of migraine headaches.

In the spinal cord enkephalins inhibit painful sensations. They react with specific receptor sites on the sensory nerve endings. They bind to opiate receptors and release controlled amounts of pain so that we are not overwhelmed by them. Enkephalin is a natural opioid. Other natural opioids are endorphins and dynorphin.

Compounds such as enkephalins which inhibit pain are eventually degraded by enzymes which are called enkephalinases. If we can prevent the breakdown of enkephalins then painful sensations are inhibited for longer.

D-phenylalanine is an amino acid which inhibits encephalin degradation. Major dietary sources are meat, fish, eggs, cheese and milk. We shall look at D-phenylalanine in more detail, later.

The morphine administered in hospital wards works on the very same opioid receptors to block pain perception.

Why does being hungry shut off the perception of pain?

Studies have shown that avoiding pain is a necessary survival skill. Research has shown that a neural pathway was activated in mice who were hungry. This inhibited the perception of and response to chronic pain.

Fasting is often recommended as it has a number of health benefits. It may be that a new health benefit is its ability to reduce pain.

Why does rubbing the affected part suppress pain?

It is an instinctive reaction to rub an injured part of the body when it is hurt. There is a good reason why we do this. Rubbing or pressing stimulates other nerve fibres and they have first choice over the nerve fibres which are transmitting pain.

This is the basis on which a TENS machine works.

Herbal Supplements which are natural painkillers

- **Alpha lipoic acid**
- **Curcumin**
- **Fish oil**
- **Ginger**
- **Resveratrol**
- **spirulina**

These supplements are considered to be natural painkillers. We will examine the composition of them to see why.

Alpha lipoic acid

Alpha-lipoic is an anti-oxidant and therefore has anti-inflammatory actions. Studies have shown that it has beneficial effects on back pain[17] although alpha-lipoic acid was also used in conjunction with gamma linoleic acid during this study.

---

[17] http://europepmc.org/abstract/med/19887043

Curcumin

Turmeric is that well known yellow spice which turns curry yellow. The active compound in turmeric is curcumin which has antioxidant and anti- inflammatory activity which helps promote healing. Studies have shown that it has pain-reducing abilities which can be as potent as over the counter medications. In clinical studies, curcumin's anti-inflammatory activity is beneficial for rheumatoid arthritis as well as a number of bowel disorders such as Crohn's disease, ulcerative colitis and irritable bowel syndrome, in addition to the inflammatory stage of OA.

There is only a small amount of curcumin in turmeric but capsules of curcumin are available at health food stores.

Ginger
Ginger has similar properties to curcumin in that it is antioxidant and anti-inflammatory in nature. However, it has to be the fresh ginger which is used, not the dried spice. Enzymes which work against inflammation are destroyed by heat so

grated ginger or thin sticks thrown into stir fries are ways in which fresh ginger can be used. Ginger is also able to help in cases of nausea which is an additional benefit over and above curcumin.

Ginger ale

Grate fresh ginger into carbonated water, add sweeteners and lemon to taste.

Fish Oil

Prostaglandins can either promote or reduce inflammation. Fish oils contain high concentrations of omega-3 fatty acids. These have been proven to shift the balance from the prostaglandins that increase inflammation to those that lessen it.

Spirulina
Spirulina is reputed to lessen the inflammatory response through anti-oxidative and anti-inflammatory mechanisms. It appears to break the cross talk between oxidative stress and inflammation.

The above are natural pain killers because they have anti-oxidative powers and are anti-inflammatory in action.

Free radicals, oxidative stress and inflammation

Free radicals are atoms or groups of atoms which have an unpaired electron. This can occur when oxygen interacts with certain molecules. These free radicals then behave a bit like an out of control pinball knocking into cells and DNA, damaging them in the process. As a result, cells may die.

Some of the degenerative disorders which can result from free radicals are
- cataracts
- Alzheimer's disease
- Certain cancers
- Accelerated aging
- Some cancers
- Heart attacks
- Arthritis

Inflammation is part of the body's natural healing process but sometimes it becomes excessive and prolonged. When this happens problems will arise. Chronic inflammation is now known to be an underlying factor in most debilitating diseases.

A vicious cycle begins when free radical damage results in inflammation. Chronic inflammation produces lots of free radicals which go onto creating more inflammation. Chronic inflammation is like an out of control forest fire in your body.

Philip Schauer, MD, director of the Bariatric and Metabolic Institute at eh Cleveland Clinic stated, 'Chronic inflammation plays a direct role in diabetes, high blood pressure, sleep apnoea, asthma and other conditions.'

Antioxidants neutralise free radicals so that they can no longer cause damage and the subsequent inflammatory response. Antioxidants effectively put a brake on chronic inflammation and prevent the insidious and uncontrolled damage that is going on inside you.

There are many antioxidants. The three main vitamins with antioxidant activity are

- Vitamin A and its precursor beta-carotene. Vitamin A is fat soluble and is found in liver, cheese, butter and oily fish. Its precursor is found in collards and orange coloured vegetables such as carrot and pumpkin.

- Vitamin C – vitamin C is found in fresh fruit and vegetables. It is water soluble and is easily destroyed by cooking. Most supermarkets have Vitamin C tablets which can be dropped into a glass of water and make a refreshing fizzy drink.

- Vitamin E – this is a fat soluble vitamin and is mainly found in nuts and wheat-germ. As high doses can cause bleeding then caution has to be applied if ibuprofen or some other NSAID is being taken alongside it as they can also create the tendency to bleed.

Vitamin C and E also work alongside each other in the brain. Vitamin E neutralises oxidants and vitamin C recycles any residue and activates it.

Vitamin E protects fatty acids in the brain, slows down neurodegeneration and the potential for microglia to develop and maintain chronic pain.

Lycopene is a bright red carotene found in tomatoes, papayas and watermelons which also has antioxidant properties.

Dark chocolate, red wine, spices such as cinnamon and nutmeg and yellow mustard seed all have antioxidant properties.

Redness and heat which occur at the site of injury are due to increased blood flow to the site of inflammation. The swelling is caused by an accumulation of fluid. This presses on nerve endings causing pain.

 Pain is also due to the release of chemicals such as bradykinin and histamine that stimulate pain receptors.

Case study

Jack was 37 and enjoyed high impact sports. He played rugby and football as well as tennis. He also enjoyed cross country running. One day on the football pitch he collided with another player. He wrenched his knee and also fractured a small

bone in his foot. Fortunately, his knee healed eventually although an x-ray showed that he had the beginnings of osteoarthritis. However, his foot did not. A small fracture was revealed on x-ray. This was dealt with appropriately at the time.

Jack, continued to be troubled by the pain in his foot. He described it as burning and painful. As a result, he had to reduce the amount of time he spent on his sports.

He was referred for a further x-ray some months later. Jack was found to have a bone spur. He was prescribed anti-inflammatories and given advice about changing his footwear so that the pressure was distributed away from the bone spur.

Magnesium as an analgesic

More and more the benefits of magnesium in relieving pain and inflammation are becoming known. Studies have found that at the cellular level, magnesium reduces inflammation. It was found that when an inflammatory condition is produced then a magnesium deficiency is created. Increasing magnesium intake decreases inflammation.

Magnesium is actively required by 700 enzyme systems in the body and there are a number of ways in which magnesium helps to reduce inflammation. Magnesium has been found to be a natural calcium channel blocker. This is important as excessive calcium is one of the most pro-inflammatory substances in the body.

The ratio of calcium to magnesium is held to be in the ratio of 800:400mg but more recent studies have argued that the amount of magnesium should equal that of calcium intake.

Dr Joseph Mercola DO has been quoted as saying

'We are all going to die at some point, but if you're deficient in magnesium you may wind up dying sooner rather than later.'

Research has shown that magnesium can be effective in both muscle and nerve pain. It is fairly clear that magnesium ameliorates muscles by its muscle relaxing abilities. It is these properties which are harnessed in the Epsom salt type bath crystals. However, a study on rats which appeared in the *Journal of Physiology* confirmed that magnesium decreases nerve pain.

N-methyl-D-aspartate (NMDA) is a pain carrying neurotransmitter. When this neurotransmitter is stimulated it is a major mechanism of pain. Some drugs such as Amantadine and Ketamine which help decrease and balance this neurotransmitter have significant side effects. For example, some of the side effects of Amantadine are listed as being:

- Depression, anxiety and irritability
- Hallucinations and confusion
- Anorexia

- Dry mouth
- Constipation
- Somnolence
- agitation

among many others.

However, magnesium has been found to calm down NMDA without the side effects that most of the prescription drugs have.

The authors of the above study have argued that magnesium deficiency can be a major amplifier of pain and have highlighted that most people are magnesium deficient.

In a rat model of osteoarthritis, a deficiency of dietary magnesium was demonstrated to enhance the amount of cartilage damage.[18]

18

https://www.ncbi.nlm.nih.gov/pmc/articles/PMC2265739/

The only contraindication to supplementing with magnesium is for those who have kidney disease

Magnesium also decreases the release of substance P and glutamate.

Substance P and glutamate are pain transmitting chemicals.

Substance P   transmits   **PAIN**
glutamate

Substance P is released from the ends of specific sensory nerves and is found in the central and peripheral nervous system. It is associated with inflammatory processes and pain.

A substance known as theanine which is found in black and green tea blocks glutamate receptors. Theanine can be obtained online or in health food shops. 200m twice daily is recommended for pain relief.

So far we have:

- Ginger blocks the production of prostaglandins.

- Ibuprofen blocks prostaglandins.

- Antihistamines block histamine release.

- Pineapple juice inhibits bradykinin

- D phenylalanine reduces pain

- Magnesium attenuates pain

Table showing common pain relieving properties and mode of action

Substance	Mode of action
fresh ginger	blocks prostaglandins
Ibuprofen	blocks prostaglandins
antihistamines	block histamine

	release
pineapple juice	Inhibits bradykinin
D phenylalanine	reduces pain
Magnesium	reduces pain

The inflammatory processes of Substance P and other inflammatory substances can therefore be addressed by over the counter medications.

Glutamate is a neurotransmitter which is associated with pain transmission. It is neurotoxic and has to be contained inside neurons. It's concentration in cells is much larger than the small amount released at crucial times. A healthy neuron only releases glutamate when it needs to pass on a message. If too much is released, pumps in the membrane suck the excess back.

When damaged cells release their glutamate the neuron isn't killed directly. The cell is excited and its pores are opened too much this allows excessive quantities of salt and calcium into the cell.

Sodium causes cell swelling which presses on adjacent blood vessels. This can ultimately lead to cell death and the release of further glutamate from damaged cells. However, this is reversible if glutamate is removed from brain fluids.

Calcium is more of a thug. If it rushes through open pores excessively it destroys the neuron's vital structures and eventually kills it. Dead cells will continue to spew out glutamate destroying areas of brain until the glutamate pumps are able to overcome the extra cellular glutamate and return it to the safety of the cell.

Alpha-Lipoic Acid – found in spinach, broccoli and liver helps glutamate transport proteins which help remove excess extracellular glutamate. [19]

The flavonoid agipenin which is found in parsley, celery, thyme, cloves, lemon balm and chamomile, among others inhibits glutamate. In culture it was found to be neuroprotective against glutamate-induced neurotoxicity in cerebellar and corticol neurons[20]. An antagonistic effect of apigenin on GABA and NMDA was found.

---

[19] http://www.jpands.org/vol9no2/blaylock.pdf
[20] https://www.ncbi.nlm.nih.gov/pubmed/15464088

GABA — gamma amino butyric acid - is a neurotransmitter which has calming and pain relieving properties. A lack of sleep which often accompanies pain can be relieved by taking 3mg of GABA about one hour before you go to bed. Most people who take GABA find themselves much calmer following it even though it is said that it does not normally cross the blood brain barrier. Some studies however, do not confirm this.

Studies have shown that people with chronic inflammatory diseases - which OA eventually becomes — have damaged pain inhibitors. That is, the pain inhibiting action of GABA becomes compromised. The pain signals which are sent to the brain via the spinal cord are practically unfiltered by GABA neurons, which are found in the spinal cord, so the pain can be felt.

Sometimes, though, the body just doesn't produce enough GABA. Further, it may not have the ability to use what it already has.

Rosmarinic acid, which is found in oregano, lemon balm, sage, marjoram and rosemary, increases

GABA levels by inhibiting an enzyme which converts GABA to L-glutamate.

A study published in the Pakistan Journal of Biological Sciences found that a salve made of ginger, cinnamon and sesame oil was just as effective as the over counter medication creams containing salicylate which is a topical analgesic.

[21]

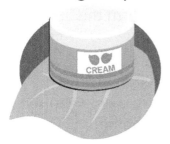

Home remedy for osteoarthritis

- Take 2 fluid ounces of Certo or some other form of pectin and add it to six ounces of red grape juice. Drink it!

---

[21] http://clipart-library.com/apply-ointment-cliparts.html

This should reduce the pain quite quickly. It is thought to work as both pectin and grape juice contain boron (an anti-inflammatory); the red grape juice contains resveratrol which also has anti-inflammatory properties.

- In the same way raisins soaked in sloe gin have also been shown to reduce the pain of osteoarthritis quite quickly.

Sloes and raisins are both packed with the mineral boron.

- The final recipe – mix half a cup of cider vinegar with four cups of apple juice and four cups of grape juice. Drink some of this, every day.

With all of the above you can add some phenylalanine to the mix (be guided by the recommended amounts on the packet). Phenylalanine can be added to drinks, yogurt, smoothies and helps relieve pain.

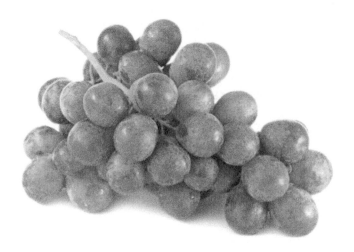

red grapes contain boron and resveratrol both of which counteract pain.

DL Phenylalanine – this essential amino acid has been well researched and documented and is effective in the control of chronic and acute pain syndromes which include

- lower back pain

- osteoarthritis

- joint pain resulting from rheumatoid arthritis

- migraine

- neuralgia

among others

DLPA appears to focus on chronic pain only. It protects the brain own natural endorphins allowing them to continue to act effectively and for longer periods than that of pharmaceutical products.

DLPA has also been found to have strong antidepressant action and is effective in relieving anxiety.

Good sources of phenylalanine are animal foods and beans and nuts. During illness when appetite is lost, and phenylalanine levels are also below optimum levels, then pain is likely to increase. Phenylalanine supplementation should be considered at this time. It is available in powdered form and is obtainable for health food shops or online.

Dosage initial dosage would be 2000mg increasing to no more than 4,500mg by two weeks. It is a good adjunctive therapy but can also be used alone.

Amino acids should always be taken on an empty stomach to maximise absorption. In free form they need no digesting and so can act within minutes – far quicker than prescribed medications unless they are the injectable form.

Glutamine is found in muscles. It is known as brain fuel as it easily passes through the blood brain barrier. Glutamine increases the amount of GABA – another amino acid and neurotransmitter - which inhibits the pain in osteoarthritis. It is the amino acid found in the intestinal gut lining and helps conditions such as Crohn's disease, leaky gut syndrome and irritable bowel syndrome. Thus it helps address gut related pain and any damage caused by NSAID's such as ibuprofen which is commonly taken by people with osteoarthritis.

The body's two primary pain modulators

The body has its own analgesic system which are the neurotransmitters. The two main ones are derived from amino acids

- Gamma amino butyric acid (GABA)

- Endorphins

It is perhaps no surprise that one of these precursor amino acids is DL phenylalanine. Seymour Ehrenpreis PhD., pharmacology professor at Chicago Medical School demonstrated that this endorphinase[22] allowed the medical school to significantly reduce the amounts of opiate medication administered.

Phenylalanine is also useful in reducing food cravings and can assist in weight loss.

.

---

[22] inhibits the breakdown of pain reliving endorphins

DMSO - this is a medicine and dietary supplement which can be taken by mouth or applied to the skin. When used topically it is used to decrease pain and speed the healing of muscle and skeletal injuries

When it is used topically it can treat painful conditions where inflammation is involved, including osteoarthritis. It is also used for foot conditions including bunions, calluses, and fungus on toenails. It has even been known to alleviate the pain from shingles.

When taken internally, it will leave the taker with garlicky smelling breath. Most people take it followed swiftly by some fruit juice, to take the taste away.

According to Hypermed Australia the consumption of DMSO should not exceed 1-2tsp daily.

Eucalyptus oil has a number of anti-inflammatory and analgesic properties. This will help to alleviate the pain of osteoarthritis. These properties of eucalyptus can be found in Vicks vapour rub which is normally bought for those with sinusitis and chesty coughs.

, **Final Thoughts**

When the root cause of pain and the different types of pain are understood then, this in itself, has the power to reduce levels of pain since it imbues a sense of power over something that once had control.

Pain is useful in telling us that something is wrong. Once we are aware of injury or illness, we are generally able to address it. Once healing has taken place then the pain should dissipate but sometimes the acute inflammatory action which is necessary for healing transforms itself into chronic inflammation.

Chronic inflammation has no useful purpose. The underlying processes in chronic inflammation begin to damage healthy tissue producing debilitating pain as they do so.

Pain is incapacitating and can reduce quality of life. However, we do have our own pain relieving mechanisms in our bodies which sometimes just need a small change in diet to be able to harness their potential

I would suggest that you go through this book again and list the treatments on a separate piece of paper. You may not decide to try them all and, indeed, the same treatments – whatever you choose - will not always work for the next person. One individual may be short of glycine and another lack vitamin D. However, if **all** the essential nutrients aren't available when the body requires them to build healthy bone and cartilage, then degeneration will occur.

I hope that this book helps in the understanding of your pain in order that you know the best way to deal with it and, in doing so, can improve the quality of your life.

Thank you for purchasing this book. Every time a book is purchased, a donation is made to one of the charities I am currently supporting. These can be found on my author's website. See below.

Other Health Related Books by the Author

- **The Reluctant Bowel**
- **A Weighty Issue**
- **Sleep, Perchance to Dream**
- **The Journey: EDS and chronic pain**
- **The MND diet: using nutrition to slow down the progress of neurodegeneration**
- **A Necessary Sorrow**
- **Treat infection Naturally**
- **Successful Aging**
- **Taking another Road: Pain: its causes and what can be done about it**
- **Osteoarthritis and Pain**
- **A Treatment Strategy for Migraine**

These can be found here on the author's page

https://www.amazon.co.uk/-/e/B07BPQZ5CD

You may also be interested in the semi-autobiographical trilogy of the authors life found in these three books

- The Prejudged
- Where the Blackbird Never Sings
- A Summer's Symphony

And the author's children's books

- Fanny and Victorian Jack
- Fanny and the Gamekeeper's Cottage

May I also make a plea that if you have enjoyed this book and benefitted from it that you would leave a review. Only one in two hundred readers, approximately, will leave a review for any book but reviews are important to authors. Thank you.

Printed in Great Britain
by Amazon

23954331R00067